DIABETIC MEAL PLANS FOR TYPE 2 DIABETES

A COMPREHENSIVE GUIDE OF CHOOSING YOUR FOOD WISELY FOR OPTIMAL BLOOD SUGAR CONTROL AND OVERALL HEALTH

Dugan Durrett

TABLE OF CONTENT

CHAPTER 1 PART 1: THE BASICS OF DIABETES FRIENDLY COOKING 12
    ESSENTIAL NUTRIENTS AND THEIR IMPACT..12
CHAPTER 2: THE DIABETES FRIENDLY PANTRY 26
    STOCKING YOUR PANTRY 26
CHAPTER 3: MEAL PLANS AND RECIPES 33
    WEEKLY MEAL PLANS.............................33
CHAPTER 4: SPECIAL CONSIDERATIONS 58
    EATING OUT AND TRAVELING 58

INTRODUCTION

Welcome to Deliciously Diabetic: A Complete Cookbook and Meal Plan for Managing Diabetes. Whether you've got currently been diagnosed or had been dwelling with diabetes for some time, this cookbook is designed to be your guide and companion in your journey towards higher fitness via delicious and nutritious meals. As someone who has walked this route, I apprehend the challenges and uncertainties that include handling diabetes. My private journey has taught me that while a diabetes diagnosis can feel overwhelming, it could additionally be an opportunity to embrace a healthier lifestyle. With the proper equipment and understanding, you can remodel your eating regimen and take manipulate of your health with out sacrificing the pleasure of ingesting.

UNDERSTANDING DIABETES

Diabetes is a continual circumstance that affects how your body approaches blood sugar (glucose). There are 3 primary types of diabetes: Type 1, Type 2, and gestational diabetes. Each kind includes specific mechanisms and control strategies, but the cornerstone of all is retaining a balanced weight loss plan.

- Type 1 Diabetes: An autoimmune circumstance wherein the body attacks insulin generating cells inside the pancreas. People with Type 1 diabetes want to take insulin and control their weight loss plan cautiously.

- Type 2 Diabetes: The maximum commonplace type, wherein the frame turns into proof against insulin or doesn't produce enough. It can often be managed through diet, exercise, and occasionally medicinal drug.

Gestational Diabetes: Occurs at some stage in being pregnant and usually is going away after childbirth, however it will increase the threat of growing Type 2 diabetes later in lifestyles.

THE ROLE OF DIET IN DIABETES MANAGEMENT

A well balanced weight reduction plan is essential in handling diabetes. By information how distinct meals have an effect on your blood sugar tiers, you may make knowledgeable selections that assist hold your blood sugar strong and decrease the threat of complications. This cookbook targets to simplify that manner by way of imparting recipes that aren't most effective diabetes friendly but also scrumptious and clean to prepare.

MYTHS AND FACTS ABOUT DIABETES AND FOOD

There are many misconceptions about what human beings with diabetes can and can't consume.

- Myth: People with diabetes want to keep away from all carbs.

- Fact: Not all carbs are created same. Complex carbohydrates like whole grains, end result, and greens are essential for a balanced weight loss program.

- Myth: Diabetics can't eat sweets or desserts.

- Fact: With right portion manage and component picks, it is viable to revel in cakes in moderation.

Myth: You need to consume special diabetic ingredients.

Fact: Healthy ingesting for diabetes is set selecting nutritious, entire foods that everybody can experience.

This cookbook is right here to manual you via these misconceptions and provide you with the know how and equipment you want to make the high quality nutritional alternatives on your health.

IMPORTANCE OF MANAGING DIABETES THROUGH DIET

Managing diabetes successfully calls for a multifaceted technique, with diet playing a pivotal function. The meals you pick to devour have a right away effect on your blood sugar tiers, typical health, and properly being.

1. Blood Sugar Control

Stable Blood Glucose Levels: The primary intention of a diabetes pleasant weight reduction plan is to maintain strong blood glucose stages. By cautiously deciding on foods which have a low glycemic index (GI) and are rich in fiber, you could prevent rapid spikes and drops in blood sugar.

Preventing Complications: Consistently excessive blood sugar levels can result in serious health complications along with cardiovascular ailment, kidney damage, nerve damage, and imaginative and prescient problems. A balanced diet helps in stopping these complications by using maintaining blood sugar inside the target range.

2. Weight Management

Healthy Weight: Maintaining a healthful weight is particularly essential for people with Type 2 diabetes, as extra weight can exacerbate insulin resistance. A diet rich in whole meals, lean proteins, and healthful fat can assist reap and keep a healthful weight.

Reducing Insulin Resistance: Weight loss, even in modest quantities, can appreciably reduce insulin resistance, making it easier in your body to modify blood sugar degrees.

3. Nutritional Balance

Essential Nutrients: A nicely balanced weight loss program ensures you acquire all of the crucial vitamins your body desires to function optimally. This consists of nutrients, minerals, antioxidants, and photochemical that help common fitness and assist control diabetes.

Energy Levels: Proper vitamins supports steady strength levels for the duration of the day, preventing the fatigue and sluggishness which could end result from negative blood sugar manage.

4. Heart Health

Cardiovascular Risk Reduction: People with diabetes are at a higher risk of growing cardiovascular illnesses. A heart healthful food regimen, low in saturated fat and high in wholesome fats, can lessen this danger. Including lots of greens, fruits, entire grains, and lean proteins facilitates hold healthful cholesterol and blood pressure degrees.

Anti inflammatory Effects: Many diabetes friendly ingredients, such as leafy greens, berries, nuts, and fatty fish, have anti inflammatory residences that guide heart health.

5. Improved Quality of Life

Enjoying Food: Managing diabetes doesn't imply you need to give up the pleasure of eating. By mastering how to put together delicious, diabetes friendly food, you may retain to enjoy numerous ingredients while coping with your situation efficiently.

Empowerment and Control: Understanding how different meals have an effect on your blood sugar tiers empowers you to make informed choices. This feel of manipulate can reduce stress and tension related to handling diabetes.

6. Preventing Longtime period Complications

Nerve and Kidney Health: High blood sugar degrees can harm nerves and kidneys over the years. A food regimen that helps blood sugar manipulate facilitates protect these vital organs from long term harm.

Eye Health: Diabetes can lead to vision troubles or even blindness. Nutrient wealthy meals that help modify blood sugar also aid eye health and help prevent diabetic retinopathy.

7. Personalized Nutrition

Tailored to Individual Needs: Everyone's body responds in a different way to meals. Working with a healthcare issuer or dietitian to broaden a personalized meal plan can help you discover what works great for your body and lifestyle.

CHAPTER 1 PART 1: THE BASICS OF DIABETES FRIENDLY COOKING

ESSENTIAL NUTRIENTS AND THEIR IMPACT

CARBOHYDRATES, PROTEINS, AND FATS: UNDERSTANDING THEIR ROLES

Managing diabetes includes understanding the jobs of the 3 major macro nutrients: carbohydrates, proteins, and fats. Each of those macro nutrients influences your blood sugar stages and average fitness in a different way.

CARBOHYDRATES

Role inside the Body:

Carbohydrates are the frame's number one source of energy. When you eat carbohydrates, your body breaks them down into glucose, which enters your bloodstream and increases your blood sugar tiers.

Types of Carbohydrates:

1. Simple Carbohydrates: Found in ingredients like sugar, sweet, and sugary liquids, these are speedy digested and may motive fast spikes in blood sugar degrees.

2. Complex Carbohydrates: Found in whole grains, legumes, veggies, and culmination, those are digested more slowly and feature a extra slow effect on blood sugar tiers because of their fiber content material.

Choosing the Right Carbohydrates:

Opt for Whole Grains: Whole grains like brown rice, quinoa, and entire wheat bread have a decrease glycemic index and are better in fiber in comparison to refined grains.

Include Plenty of Vegetables: Non starchy greens like leafy veggies, broccoli, and peppers are low in carbohydrates and excessive in nutrients.

 Moderate Fruit Intake: Choose culmination which might be decrease in sugar and higher in fiber, which includes berries, apples, and pears.

Portion Control:

Even healthy carbohydrates can affect blood sugar stages if consumed in massive quantities. Use element control to control your consumption and distribute your carbohydrate intake lightly for the duration of the day.

2. Glycemic Index and Glycemic Load

 Explanation and importance for diabetes.

 Carbohydrates, Proteins, and Fats:

Explanation and Importance for Diabetes

CARBOHYDRATES

Role in the Body:

Carbohydrates are the primary source of strength for the frame. They are broken down into glucose at some point of digestion, which enters the bloodstream and increases blood sugar levels.

TYPES OF CARBOHYDRATES:

1. Simple Carbohydrates: These include sugars observed in chocolates, sugary drinks, and processed meals. They are quickly digested and might cause rapid spikes in blood sugar levels.

2. Complex Carbohydrates: These encompass starches and fibers discovered in whole grains, legumes, vegetables, and fruits. They are digested greater slowly, leading to a gradual upward thrust in blood sugar stages.

IMPORTANCE FOR DIABETES:

Blood Sugar Management: For individuals with diabetes, handling carbohydrate consumption is important. Monitoring the sort and amount of carbohydrates consumed allows save you spikes and dips in blood sugar stages.

 Glycemic Index (GI): Choosing low GI ingredients, inclusive of whole grains and non starchy vegetables, can assist keep solid blood sugar degrees. Low GI foods are digested and absorbed more slowly, inflicting a slower rise in blood sugar.

 Fiber: High fiber meals are mainly beneficial as they assist regulate blood sugar stages, improve digestion, and growth satiety, which could aid in weight management.

3. Reading Food Labels

Understanding nutritional data.

Identifying Hidden Sugars and Unhealthy Fats

Managing diabetes efficiently includes being vigilant approximately hidden sugars and bad fat for your weight reduction plan. Both could have big affects on blood sugar stages, coronary heart health, and ordinary nicely being.

 Hidden Sugars

Sources of Hidden Sugars:

Hidden sugars are delivered sugars that aren't constantly apparent in processed and packaged ingredients. They can be found in:

 Condiments: Ketchup, barbeque sauce, salad dressings, and marinades regularly contain delivered sugars.

 Beverages: Sodas, fruit juices, flavored waters, electricity beverages, or even a few kinds of flavored espresso and tea.

 Snack Foods: Granola bars, flavored yogurt, cereals, and snack cakes.

 Baked Goods: Bread, pastries, truffles, and cookies.

 Processed Foods: Canned soups, pasta sauces, and prepared made food.

Reading Food Labels:

1. Check the Ingredients List: Look for phrases that suggest introduced sugars, consisting of sucrose, high fructose corn syrup, cane sugar, maltose, dextrose, and honey.

2. Nutrition Facts: Look on the "Total Sugars" and "Added Sugars" at the nutrients label. Aim for ingredients with little to no delivered sugars.

3. Recognize Sugar Alternatives: Be privy to sugar alcohols and non nutritive sweeteners (e.G., aspartame, sucralose, stevia), which may also impact blood sugar levels in a different way.

AVOIDING HIDDEN SUGARS:

Choose Whole Foods: Opt for sparkling, entire foods over processed ones.

Make Your Own: Prepare self made variations of condiments, snacks, and food to control the components.

Limit Sugary Beverages: Drink water, unsweetened tea, or coffee instead of sugary drinks.

IDENTIFYING HIDDEN SUGARS AND UNHEALTHY FATS

Managing diabetes entails being aware of hidden sugars and unhealthy fats in your eating regimen, as each can impact blood sugar tiers and average health negatively.

Hidden Sugars

Sources of Hidden Sugars:

Hidden sugars are frequently brought to processed meals to enhance flavor. They can be determined in:

Condiments: Ketchup, barbecue sauce, salad dressings, and marinades.

Beverages: Sodas, fruit juices, electricity beverages, flavored waters, and some sorts of espresso and tea.

Snack Foods: Granola bars, flavored yogurt, cereal, and sweetened nut butters.

Baked Goods: Cookies, desserts, pastries, and desserts.

Processed Foods: Canned soups, sauces, and geared up to consume meals.

Tips for Identifying Hidden Sugars:

1. Read Ingredient Lists: Look for terms indicating brought sugars such as sucrose, high fructose corn syrup, cane sugar, maltose, dextrose, and honey.

2. Check Nutrition Labels: Review the "Total Sugars" and "Added Sugars" sections. Choose products with minimal introduced sugars or choose those categorised as "no added sugars."

3. Be Cautious with Sugar Substitutes: Sugar alcohols (e.G., sorbitol, xylitol) and synthetic sweeteners (e.G., aspartame, saccharin) may have minimum effect on blood sugar however can motive digestive issues in some humans.

Strategies to Reduce Hidden Sugars:

Choose Whole Foods: Opt for fresh fruits and vegetables, lean proteins, and complete grains.

Prepare Meals at Home: Cook from scratch to govern sugar content material.

Drink Water: Avoid sugary drinks; drink water, herbal teas, or unsweetened espresso instead.

Read Labels Carefully: Even seemingly healthy products may also include hidden sugars.

MEAL PLANNING FOR DIABETES

Creating balanced food.

Creating balanced food is essential for coping with diabetes efficaciously and promoting overall fitness. A balanced meal consists of a mixture of carbohydrates, proteins, healthy fats, fiber, and crucial nutrients.

Principles for Creating Balanced Meals

1. Include Lean Protein

Proteins are important for retaining muscle tissues, helping immune function, and stabilizing blood sugar stages. Choose lean sources of protein which includes:

Skinless rooster

Fish and seafood

Lean cuts of beef or beef

Tofu, tempeh, or other plant based totally proteins

Beans, lentils, and legumes

2. Choose Complex Carbohydrates

Complex carbohydrates are digested extra slowly, main to a gradual upward push in blood sugar tiers. They additionally provide vital nutrients and fiber. Opt for:

Whole grains like brown rice, quinoa, whole wheat pasta, and oats

Non starchy vegetables which includes leafy veggies, broccoli, cauliflower, peppers, and tomatoes

Fresh fruits like berries, apples, pears, and citrus end result

3. Incorporate Healthy Fats

- Healthy fat are critical for heart health and may assist improve insulin sensitivity. Include sources of monounsaturated and polyunsaturated fat which includes:
- Avocados
- Nuts and seeds (almonds, walnuts, chia seeds, flax seeds)
- Olive oil, avocado oil, and canola oil
- Fatty fish like salmon, trout, and sardines

4. Add Fiber Rich Foods

Fiber allows alter blood sugar tiers, promotes satiety, and helps digestive health. Include excessive fiber meals including:

Whole grains (specially people with intact grains)

Beans, lentils, and legumes

Nuts and seeds

Vegetables (in particular non starchy greens)

5. Control Portions

- Managing portion sizes is essential for controlling blood sugar tiers and handling weight. Use the plate technique as a manual:

- Fill 1/2 of your plate with non starchy greens.

- Divide the alternative half among lean protein and complex carbohydrates.

- Add a serving of healthful fats along with a drizzle of olive oil or a handful of nuts.

6. Watch Sodium and Added Sugars

Limiting sodium and heading off delivered sugars can assist reduce the danger of cardiovascular headaches. Choose low sodium options and limit delivered sugars by cooking from scratch and analyzing meals labels cautiously.

7. Consider Meal Timing and Frequency

Spacing food flippantly at some stage in the day (e.G., breakfast, lunch, dinner, and snacks) can assist regulate blood sugar ranges. Avoid skipping food and purpose for consistency in meal timing to aid solid electricity tiers.

CHAPTER 2: THE DIABETES FRIENDLY PANTRY

STOCKING YOUR PANTRY

Must have components.

To create balanced and diabetes friendly meals, it is useful to inventory your kitchen with vital ingredients that offer nutritional blessings whilst supporting you manipulate blood sugar degrees effectively.

Pantry Staples:

1. Whole Grains:

- Brown rice
- Quinoa
- Whole wheat pasta
- Rolled oats

2. Legumes and Beans:

- Lentils
- Black beans
- Chickpeas

- Kidney beans

3. Healthy Cooking Oils:

- Olive oil
- Avocado oil
- Canola oil

4. Nuts and Seeds:

- Almonds
- Walnuts
- Chia seeds
- Flaxseeds

5. Nut Butters:

- Natural peanut butter
- Almond butter

6. Herbs and Spices:

- Cinnamon
- Turmeric
- Garlic powder
- Basil
- Oregano
- Paprika

7. Vinegars:

Balsamic vinegar

Apple cider vinegar

Red wine vinegar

8. Canned Tomatoes and Tomato Paste:

(Low sodium variations if viable)

9. Low Sodium Broth or Stock: (Vegetable, hen, or pork)

10. Whole Wheat Flour or Almond Flour: (For baking and cooking)

Refrigerator Essentials:

1. Lean Proteins:

Skinless bird breasts

Turkey breast

- Lean cuts of red meat or beef
- Fish (salmon, trout, tilapia)

2. Fresh Vegetables:

- Leafy greens (spinach, kale, arugula)
- Broccoli
- Bell peppers
- Zucchini

- Cauliflower

- Tomatoes

HOW TO TASTE FOOD WITHOUT BROUGHT SUGARS OR DANGEROUS FATS.

Flavoring food without relying on added sugars or dangerous fats is not best feasible but can also beautify the herbal taste of substances while keeping your food nutritious and diabetes pleasant.

1. Herbs and Spices

Benefits: Herbs and spices upload intensity and complexity to dishes without adding extra calories, sugars, or bad fat. They are also rich in antioxidants and can have fitness selling properties.

Examples:

- Basil: Fresh or dried, provides a candy, barely peppery flavor.

- Cinnamon: Adds warm temperature and sweetness, first rate for oatmeal or baked goods.
- Turmeric: Earthy taste with anti inflammatory properties, best for curries.
- Garlic powder: Intense flavor with out the want for brought salt or fat.
- Paprika: Adds a moderate warmness and vibrant coloration to dishes.

2. Citrus Juices and Zest

Benefits: Citrus end result like lemon, lime, and orange offer a burst of freshness and acidity that enhances flavors with out additional sugars or fat.

Examples:

Lemon juice: Adds brightness to salads, fish, and veggies.

- Lime zest: Grated lime peel provides a tangy aroma to marinades and dressings.

- Orange segments: Adds sweetness and acidity to savory dishes like salads or chicken marinades.

3. Vinegars

Benefits: Vinegars such as balsamic, apple cider, and purple wine vinegar upload tanginess and intensity to dishes with out sugar or unhealthy fats. They can be utilized in dressings, marinades, and sauces.

Examples:

Balsamic vinegar: Sweet and tangy, terrific for drizzling over roasted greens or salads.

Apple cider vinegar: Adds a tart taste to marinades and pickled vegetables.

Red wine vinegar: Adds a robust flavor to marinades and vinaigrette.

4. Natural Sweeteners in Moderation

Benefits: If a touch of sweetness is favored, herbal sweeteners like stevia or monk fruit can be used sparingly. They are low in energy and do now not appreciably effect blood sugar tiers.

Examples:

Stevia: A plant based sweetener that can be used in liquids or desserts.

Monk fruit extract: Provides sweetness without energy, appropriate for baking or sweetening sauces.

5. Aromatics like Onions and Garlic

Benefits: Onions and garlic upload savory intensity and complexity to dishes. They may be sauteed or roasted to decorate their herbal sweetness without adding unhealthy fat.

Examples:

- Onions: Sauteed onions add sweetness to soups, stews, and sauces.
- Garlic: Roasted garlic cloves can be mashed and used as a spread or introduced to dressings and marinades.

CHAPTER 3: MEAL PLANS AND RECIPES

WEEKLY MEAL PLANS

four weeks of meal plans for breakfast, lunch, dinner, and snacks.

Creating a balanced and diabetes friendly meal plan for four weeks includes range, vitamins, and delicious flavors.

Week 1

Day 1

- Breakfast: Greek yogurt with berries and a sprinkle of chia seeds
- Lunch: Quinoa salad with grilled chicken, blended veggies, cherry tomatoes, and balsamic vinaigrette
- Dinner: Baked salmon with roasted sweet potatoes and steamed broccoli
- Snack: Apple slices with almond butter

Day 2

- Breakfast: Spinach and feta omelet with entire wheat toast
- Lunch: Lentil soup with a facet salad (combined vegetables, cucumber, bell peppers)
- Dinner: Stir fried tofu with combined greens (bell peppers, broccoli, carrots) and brown rice
- Snack: Mixed nuts (almonds, walnuts) and a small orange

Day 3

- Breakfast: Overnight oats with almond milk, topped with sliced bananas and a sprinkle of cinnamon
- Lunch: Grilled vegetable wrap with hummus in a whole wheat tortilla
- Dinner: Turkey chili with kidney beans, served with a side of roasted Brussels sprouts
- Snack: Carrot sticks with tzatziki dip

Day 4

- Breakfast: Smoothie bowl with spinach, berries, almond milk, and a handful of granola
- Lunch: Chicken and vegetable stir fry (zucchini, bell peppers, snap peas) over quinoa
- Dinner: Baked cod with a side of quinoa pilaf and steamed asparagus
- Snack: Cottage cheese with pineapple chunks

Day 5

- Breakfast: Whole grain toast with avocado spread and poached eggs
- Lunch: Greek salad with grilled shrimp, olives, feta cheese, and a lemon oregano dressing
- Dinner: Spaghetti squash with marinara sauce, lean floor turkey, and a aspect of roasted cauliflower
- Snack: Edamame (steamed soybeans)

Day 6

- Breakfast: Scrambled eggs with sauteed spinach and complete grain toast
- Lunch: Quinoa and black bean crammed peppers with a facet of combined greens
- Dinner: Grilled bird breast with roasted sweet potato wedges and green beans
- Snack: Greek yogurt with a drizzle of honey and sliced strawberries

Day 7

Breakfast: Chia seed pudding with unsweetened almond milk, crowned with sparkling mango

Lunch: Turkey and avocado wrap in an entire wheat tortilla, served with a facet of cucumber slices

BREAK FAST RECIPES

Smoothies and shakes.

Smoothies and shakes may be top notch alternatives for breakfast, snacks, or maybe a mild meal, especially when dealing with diabetes. They may be packed with nutrients, fiber, and protein at the same time as being low in introduced sugars.

EGG DISHES.

Egg dishes may be versatile, pleasant, and nutritious options for breakfast, lunch, or dinner, specially for those managing diabetes.

1. Veggie Omelet

Ingredients:

- 2 eggs
- 1/4 cup diced bell peppers (any coloration)
- 1/4 cup diced tomatoes
- 1/four cup chopped spinach
- Salt and pepper to taste
- 1 tsp olive oil

Diabetic pleasant pancakes and waffles.

Diabetic pleasant pancakes and waffles may be delicious and pleasant with out causing large spikes in blood sugar stages.

TIPS FOR DIABETIC FRIENDLY PANCAKES AND WAFFLES

1. Choose Whole Grains: Opt for whole grain flours like whole wheat flour, oat flour, or almond flour in preference to refined white flour. Whole grains have a lower glycemic index and offer more fiber, which enables alter blood sugar stages.

2. Use Natural Sweeteners Sparingly: Instead of sugar, use small quantities of natural sweeteners like mashed ripe bananas, unsweetened applesauce, or a small quantity of honey or maple syrup. Alternatively, you may use sugar substitutes like stevia or monk fruit sweetener.

3. Add Protein: Adding protein in your pancakes or waffles can help stabilize blood sugar levels and preserve you feeling complete longer. You can incorporate protein powder (ideally unsweetened), Greek yogurt, or almond meal into the batter.

3. Lunch Recipes

Salads and dressings.

Creating diabetes pleasant salads and dressings includes specializing in nutrient dense components, controlling element sizes, and using dressings which are low in added sugars and dangerous fat.

DIABETES FRIENDLY SALADS

Salad Ingredients:

- Leafy Greens: Spinach, kale, arugula, romaine lettuce
- Non Starchy Vegetables: Cucumbers, bell peppers, tomatoes, carrots, broccoli
- Protein: Grilled bird breast, salmon, tofu, chickpeas, hard boiled eggs
- Healthy Fats: Avocado, nuts (almonds, walnuts), seeds (chia seeds, flax seeds)
- Whole Grains: Quinoa, brown rice, farro (in moderation)

Salad Dressing Ideas

1. Balsamic Vinaigrette:

- 2 tbsp balsamic vinegar

- 1 tbsp olive oil

- 1 tsp Dijon mustard

- half of tsp honey (elective)

- Salt and pepper to flavor

SOUPS AND STEWS.

Soups and stews may be comforting, nutritious, and diabetes friendly when organized with healthful components and conscious of their impact on blood sugar stages.

Tips for Diabetes Friendly Soups and Stews

1. Choose Lean Proteins: Opt for lean cuts of meat (like chicken breast or turkey), seafood, or plant based totally proteins (consisting of beans or lentils) to add protein without immoderate fat.

2. Load Up on Vegetables: Use a number of colourful, non starchy veggies like spinach, kale, carrots, celery, bell peppers, and

tomatoes. Vegetables upload fiber and crucial vitamins without significantly impacting blood sugar tiers.

3. Use Whole Grains Sparingly: If including grains like barley, quinoa, or brown rice, achieve this in moderation to hold carbohydrate levels in test. These grains provide fiber however can have an effect on blood sugar levels, so component manage is prime.

SANDWICHES AND WRAPS.

Sandwiches and wraps may be flexible, enjoyable, and diabetes pleasant with the right ingredients and portion sizes.

Tips for Diabetes Friendly Sandwiches and Wraps

CHOOSE WHOLE GRAIN BREAD OR WRAPS:

Opt for entire grain options like complete wheat bread, complete grain wraps, or sprouted grain bread. These choices provide greater fiber and feature a decrease glycemic index in comparison to subtle white bread.

INCLUDE LEAN PROTEINS:

Choose lean protein sources which includes grilled bird breast, turkey, tuna, lean roast beef, or tofu. Protein enables preserve you complete and stabilizes blood sugar ranges.

ADD PLENTY OF VEGETABLES:

- Load up your sandwich or wrap with clean vegetables which includes lettuce, spinach, tomatoes, cucumbers, bell peppers, and onions.

DINNER RECIPES

Poultry, meat, and fish dishes.

Creating diabetes pleasant chicken, meat, and fish dishes involves specializing in lean cuts of meat, incorporating lots of vegetables, and the usage of healthy cooking methods.

- Poultry Dishes

- Grilled Chicken with Quinoa and Roasted Vegetables
- Ingredients:
- Skinless chook breasts
- Quinoa

Assorted vegetables (bell peppers, zucchini, carrots)

Olive oil

Garlic powder, salt, and pepper

Instructions:

1. Marinate fowl breasts with olive oil, garlic powder, salt, and pepper.

2. Grill hen till fully cooked.

Three. Cook quinoa consistent with bundle instructions.

Four. Roast greens tossed with olive oil, salt, and pepper.

5. Serve grilled chook over a mattress of quinoa with roasted greens on the side.

Meat Dishes

Lean Beef Stir Fry with Brown Rice

Ingredients:

Lean pork (inclusive of sirloin or flank steak), thinly sliced

Mixed vegetables (broccoli, snap peas, bell peppers)

PLANT BASED TOTALLY DINNERS.

Plant based dinners may be delicious, pleasant, and useful for dealing with diabetes by means of that specialize in complete ingredients wealthy in fiber, nutrients, and minerals.

1. Quinoa Stuffed Bell Peppers

Ingredients:

- Bell peppers (any coloration)
- Quinoa
- Black beans
- Corn kernels
- Diced tomatoes
- Onion, diced
- Garlic, minced

Cumin, paprika, salt, and pepper to flavor

Olive oil

Instructions:

1. Preheat oven to 375°F (one hundred ninety°C).

2. Cook quinoa according to bundle instructions.

Three. Cut the tops off bell peppers and cast off seeds and membranes.

Four. In a skillet, heat olive oil over medium warmth. Add onion and garlic, saute until softened.

Five. Stir in black beans, corn, diced tomatoes, cooked quinoa, and seasonings. Cook for 57 mins until heated through.

6. Stuff the bell peppers with the quinoa combination and area them in a baking dish.

SNACK RECIPES

Healthy and brief snack thoughts.

Healthy and short snack ideas are important, in particular for handling diabetes, to keep

blood sugar levels strong and offer lasting
energy.

1. Greek Yogurt with Berries

- Plain Greek yogurt topped with
  sparkling berries (such as strawberries,
  blueberries, or raspberries)

- Optional: Sprinkle with a small amount
  of nuts or seeds for delivered crunch and
  wholesome fats.

2. Sliced Veggies with Hummus

- Assorted clean veggies (carrots,
  cucumber, bell peppers) sliced into
  sticks or rounds

- Serve with a part of hummus for
  dipping. Hummus affords protein and
  fiber, even as veggies are low in energy
  and full of nutrients.

3. Apple Slices with Almond Butter

- Crisp apple slices paired with natural
  almond butter (look for sorts without
  brought sugars or oils)

- Almond butter presents healthful fat and protein, at the same time as apples provide fiber and herbal sweetness.

4. Hard Boiled Eggs

Prepare a batch of tough boiled eggs in advance of time for short snacks at some point of the week.

Eggs are a splendid supply of protein and essential nutrients. Sprinkle with a pinch of salt and pepper if preferred.

5. Cottage Cheese with Pineapple

Low fat cottage cheese crowned with clean pineapple chunks

Cottage cheese is high in protein and low in carbohydrates, whilst pineapple adds natural sweetness and nutrition C.

6. Mixed Nuts

A handful of unsalted blended nuts, including almonds, walnuts, and pistachios

Nuts are wealthy in healthful fat, protein, and fiber, offering a satisfying snack that helps maintain you full.

7. Rice Cake with Avocado

Lightly salted rice cake topped with mashed avocado

Avocado offers healthy fat and fiber, while the rice cake offers a crunchy base.

8. Cucumber and Tomato Salad

Sliced cucumber and cherry tomatoes tossed with a drizzle of olive oil, balsamic vinegar, and a sprinkle of fresh herbs (like basil or parsley)

This clean snack is low in energy and carbohydrates but rich in nutrients and antioxidants.

HOMEMADE DIABETIC FRIENDLY BARS AND BITES.

Creating home made diabetic pleasant bars and bites permits you to control the ingredients, ensuring they may be nutritious and low in delivered sugars.

1. Nut and Seed Bars

Ingredients:

1 cup blended nuts (almonds, walnuts, cashews)

1/2 cup seeds (pumpkin seeds, sunflower seeds)

half cup unsweetened shredded coconut

half of cup almond butter or peanut butter (herbal, no introduced sugars)

1/four cup honey or maple syrup (non compulsory, regulate to taste)

half of tsp vanilla extract

Pinch of salt

Optional addins: dark chocolate chips, dried fruit (like cranberries or raisins)

Instructions:

1. In a food processor, pulse the nuts, seeds, and shredded coconut until coarsely chopped.

2. In a saucepan, warmth almond butter (or peanut butter), honey (or maple syrup), vanilla extract, and salt over low heat until nicely blended and slightly melted.

3. Pour the nut and seed combination into the saucepan with the almond butter mixture. Stir till frivolously lined.

4. Press the combination firmly into a lined baking dish or pan.

5. Optional: Sprinkle with darkish chocolate chips or dried fruit and press them into the aggregate.

6. Refrigerate for at the least 2 hours till organization. Cut into bars or squares.

NUT AND SEED MIXES.

Nut and seed mixes make top notch diabetes friendly snacks, supplying a great stability of wholesome fats, protein, and fiber, which can help stabilize blood sugar degrees. Here are a few hints for creating your personal mixes, along side some recipe thoughts:

TIPS FOR CREATING NUT AND SEED MIXES

1. Choose a Variety of Nuts and Seeds: Include different sorts to maximize dietary blessings. Good options encompass almonds, walnuts, pecans, cashews, pistachios, sunflower seeds, pumpkin seeds, chia seeds, and flax seeds.

2. Avoid Added Sugars and Excessive Salt: Use uncooked or lightly roasted nuts and seeds with out delivered sugars or immoderate salt. You can roast them yourself to manipulate the seasoning.

6. Dessert Recipes

Low sugar and sugar loose desserts.

Creating low sugar and sugar free cakes can fulfill your sweet enamel without causing huge spikes in blood sugar tiers.

1. Chia Seed Pudding

Ingredients:

1/four cup chia seeds

1 cup unsweetened almond milk (or every other milk of choice)

1 tsp vanilla extract

12 tbsp sugar unfastened sweetener (inclusive of stevia or monk fruit sweetener)

Fresh berries for topping

Instructions:

1. In a bowl, mix chia seeds, almond milk, vanilla extract, and sweetener.

2. Stir well to mix and let it sit down for five mins.

Three. Stir once more to save you clumping, then cowl and refrigerate for at least 2 hours or overnight.

4. Serve chilled, topped with sparkling berries.

2. Avocado Chocolate Mousse

Ingredients:

2 ripe avocados

1/4 cup unsweetened cocoa powder

1/4 cup almond milk

23 tbsp sugar free sweetener

1 tsp vanilla extract

FRUIT PRIMARILY BASED TREATS.

Fruit primarily based treats may be a fresh and healthy way to experience dessert even as handling diabetes.

1. Baked Apples

Ingredients:

4 medium apples (which include Granny Smith or Honey crisp)

1/four cup chopped nuts (walnuts, pecans)

1/4 cup raisins or dried cranberries (elective)

1 tsp floor cinnamon

1/2 tsp floor nutmeg

1/four cup water

Diabetic pleasant baking recipes.

Baking can still be part of a diabetes friendly weight reduction plan with some considerate component swaps and recipe adjustments.

1. Almond Flour Blueberry Muffins

Ingredients:

2 cups almond flour

half of tsp baking soda

1/four tsp salt

3 huge eggs

1/4 cup unsweetened almond milk

1/four cup sugar loose sweetener (along with erythritol or stevia)

1 tsp vanilla extract

1 cup sparkling or frozen blueberries

BEVERAGE RECIPES

Infused waters.

Infused waters are a refreshing and healthy manner to live hydrated even as adding a chunk of flavor with out introduced sugars.

TIPS FOR MAKING INFUSED WATERS

1. Use Fresh Ingredients: Fresh culmination, vegetables, and herbs provide the quality flavor and nutritional blessings.

2. Slice Thinly: Thin slices launch extra taste into the water.

3. Let It Steep: Allow the components to steep in the water for at least 2 hours, or overnight for a stronger flavor.

4. Experiment with Combinations: Mix one of a kind fruits, greens, and herbs to discover your favorite flavors.

DIABETIC PLEASANT SMOOTHIES AND JUICES

Diabetic pleasant smoothies and juices may be a super way to experience fresh flavors while dealing with blood sugar stages.

Tips for Diabetes Friendly Smoothies and Juices

1. Choose Low Glycemic Fruits: Opt for fruits like berries, apples, pears, and citrus culmination which have a decrease impact on blood sugar.

2. Add Protein and Healthy Fats: Include components like Greek yogurt, protein powder, nuts, seeds, or avocado to assist stability blood sugar.

3. Limit Added Sugars: Avoid including sugars or excessive sugar culmination like bananas, mangoes, and pineapples.

4. Incorporate Vegetables: Adding leafy veggies, cucumbers, or carrots can raise nutrition with out including many carbs.

5. Use Unsweetened Liquid Bases: Opt for unsweetened almond milk, coconut water, or simply plain water.

Low carb coffee and tea options.

Low carb espresso and tea alternatives can be each pleasurable and diabetes pleasant.

Low Carb Coffee Options

1. Black Coffee

Ingredients: Freshly brewed espresso

Instructions: Enjoy black espresso warm or iced, without including sugar. If you decide upon a sweeter taste, use a sugar loose sweetener like stevia or monk fruit.

2. Bulletproof Coffee

Ingredients:

- 1 cup brewed espresso
- 12 tbsp unsalted butter or ghee
- 1 tbsp coconut oil or MCT oil

Instructions:

- 1. Brew a cup of coffee.
- 2. Blend the coffee with butter and coconut oil until frothy.

3. Almond Milk Latte

Ingredients:

1 cup unsweetened almond milk

1 shot espresso or 1/2 cup sturdy brewed coffee

Sugar loose sweetener (optional)

Instructions:

1. Heat almond milk until heat.

2. Froth the almond milk the use of a milk frothier or whisk.

3. Pour the coffee or espresso right into a mug and top with frothed almond milk.

4. Sweeten with a sugar free sweetener if favored.

CHAPTER 4: SPECIAL CONSIDERATIONS

EATING OUT AND TRAVELING

TIPS FOR MAKING WHOLESOME ALTERNATIVES AT EATING PLACES. Packing diabetes pleasant snacks and food for journey permit you to preserve healthy eating habits and control blood sugar degrees on the pass.

Tips for Packing Travel Snacks and Meals

1. Plan Ahead: Prepare snacks and food earlier to ensure you have got healthful alternatives to be had.

2. Use Insulated Containers: Use insulated lunch luggage and ice packs to keep perishable objects sparkling.

3. Opt for Non Perishables: Include some nonperishable objects that don't require refrigeration.

4. Balance Nutrients: Aim for a combination of protein, healthful fat, and fiber to keep you complete and maintain regular blood sugar tiers.

5. Stay Hydrated: Pack a refillable water bottle to stay hydrated.

SNACK IDEAS

1. Nuts and Seeds Mix: A mix of almonds, walnuts, sunflower seeds, and pumpkin seeds.

2. Fresh Fruit: Apples, berries, or small oranges. Pair with a handful of nuts or a small piece of cheese for balance.

3. Vegetable Sticks: Carrot sticks, cucumber slices, and bell pepper strips with hummus.

4. Cheese: Individually wrapped cheese sticks or slices.

5. Hard Boiled Eggs: Precooked and peeled, stored in a cooler.

6. Greek Yogurt: Individual servings of plain Greek yogurt with a small portion of clean berries or a sprinkle of nuts.

7. Whole Grain Crackers: Paired with nut butter or low sodium canned tuna.

MEAL IDEAS

1. Chicken and Veggie Wraps:

- Whole grain or low carb wraps with grilled fowl, spinach, sliced bell peppers, and a mild dressing or hummus.

2. Quinoa Salad:

- Quinoa mixed with chopped greens, chickpeas, and a lemon French dressing.

3. Tuna Salad Lettuce Wraps:

- Tuna salad made with Greek yogurt or avocado, wrapped in huge lettuce leaves.

2. Cooking for the Family

- Making diabetes friendly meals that everybody will love.

Creating diabetes friendly meals that everyone will love entails that specialize in complete, nutritious components and scrumptious flavors.

TIPS FOR DIABETES FRIENDLY MEALS

1. Focus on Whole Foods: Use sparkling vegetables, lean proteins, complete grains, and wholesome fat.

2. Control Portions: Balance your plate with appropriate quantities of carbohydrates, proteins, and fats.

Three. Limit Added Sugars and Refined Carbs: Use natural sweeteners and entire grains instead of processed sugars and subtle carbohydrates.

4. Incorporate Fiber: Fiber allows manage blood sugar levels and continues you complete longer.

5. Flavor with Herbs and Spices: Enhance dishes with fresh herbs, spices, and citrus in place of counting on sugar and salt.

Recipes

1. Grilled Lemon Herb Chicken with Quinoa and Vegetables

Ingredients:

- four boneless, skinless hen breasts
- 1/four cup olive oil
- 2 lemons (one for juice and zest, one sliced)
- three cloves garlic, minced
- 1 tsp dried oregano
- 1 tsp dried thyme
- Salt and pepper to taste
- 1 cup quinoa
- 2 cups low sodium bird broth
- 1 cup cherry tomatoes, halved
- 1 cucumber, diced
- 1/four cup fresh parsley, chopped

Instructions:

1. Marinate Chicken:

- In a bowl, whisk collectively olive oil, lemon juice and zest, garlic, oregano, thyme, salt, and pepper.
- Add hen breasts and marinate for as a minimum half hour.

2. Cook Quinoa:

- Rinse quinoa below bloodless water.
- In a pot, convey chicken broth to a boil. Add quinoa, reduce warmness, cowl, and simmer for 15 mins or till liquid is absorbed.

3. Grill Chicken:

- Preheat grill to medium high heat.
- Grill chook for six7 minutes on each facet or until absolutely cooked. Grill lemon slices alongside for garnish.

4. Assemble Plate:

- Fluff quinoa with a fork and blend in cherry tomatoes, cucumber, and parsley.

- Serve grilled hen over the quinoa salad, garnished with grilled lemon slices.

2. Vegetable StirFry with Tofu

Ingredients:

- 1 block company tofu, drained and cubed
- 2 tbsp soy sauce (low sodium)
- 1 tbsp sesame oil
- 2 cloves garlic, minced
- 1 tbsp fresh ginger, grated
- 1 bell pepper, sliced
- 1 broccoli crown, reduce into florets
- 1 carrot, thinly sliced
- 1 cup snap peas
- 2 inexperienced onions, sliced
- 1/4 cup vegetable broth
- 1 tbsp cornstarch (non compulsory, for thickening)
- Cooked brown rice or cauliflower rice for serving

Instructions:

1. Prepare Tofu:

- Press tofu to cast off excess moisture. Cube and marinate in 1 tbsp soy sauce for 10 minutes.

2. StirFry Veggies:

- Heat sesame oil in a large skillet or wok over medium high heat.
- Add garlic and ginger, saute for 1 minute.
- Add bell pepper, broccoli, carrot, and snap peas. Stir fry till vegetables are tender crisp.

3. Cook Tofu:

Push greens to the side and add tofu to the skillet. Cook till golden brown on all aspects.

4. Combine and Thicken:

- Mix remaining soy sauce with vegetable broth (and cornstarch if the usage of) and pour over stir fry. Stir till sauce thickens.

5. Serve:

- Serve stir fry over cooked brown rice or cauliflower rice, topped with sliced inexperienced onions.

3. Baked Salmon with Asparagus and Sweet Potatoes

Ingredients:

- 4 salmon fillets
- 1 bunch asparagus, trimmed
- 2 medium sweet potatoes, cubed
- 2 tbsp olive oil
- 1 lemon, thinly sliced
- 3 cloves garlic, minced
- Salt and pepper to flavor
- Fresh dill or parsley for garnish

Instructions:

1. Preheat Oven:

Preheat oven to four hundred°F (200°C).

2. Prepare Sweet Potatoes:

- Toss candy potato cubes with 1 tbsp olive oil, salt, and pepper. Spread on a baking sheet and roast for 20 minutes.

3. Prepare Salmon and Asparagus:

- Season salmon fillets with salt and pepper. Place on a baking sheet covered with lemon slices.

- Toss asparagus with final olive oil, garlic, salt, and pepper. Add to the baking sheet with salmon.

4. Bake:

- Bake salmon and asparagus for 1520 mins, or till salmon is cooked via and asparagus is soft.

5. Serve:

- Serve salmon fillets with roasted candy potatoes and asparagus, garnished with sparkling dill or parsley.

3. Managing Blood Sugar Levels

TIPS FOR TRACKING AND MAINTAINING HEALTHY BLOOD SUGAR LEVELS.

Monitoring and maintaining healthy blood sugar stages is important for dealing with diabetes effectively.

1. Regular Monitoring

Use a Glucose Meter:

- Frequency: Test your blood sugar stages as encouraged by means of your healthcare company. This can also consist of checking out earlier than and after meals, before mattress, and all through bodily pastime.

- Record: Keep a log of your blood sugar readings, consisting of the date, time, and any notes about meals, exercising, or pressure levels.

Continuous Glucose Monitoring (CGM):

Device: Consider the use of a CGM device that tracks blood sugar ranges at some point of the day and night, supplying actual time statistics and indicators for high or low degrees.

2. Balanced Diet

Carbohydrate Counting:

- Track Carbs: Be conscious of your carbohydrate intake. Use food labels, apps, or assets to be counted carbs appropriately.

- Spread Intake: Distribute your carbohydrate intake evenly at some stage in the day to keep away from spikes in blood sugar.

Choose Low Glycemic Foods:

- Low GI Foods: Opt for ingredients with a low glycemic index (GI), along with entire grains, legumes, non starchy vegetables, and maximum end result.

- Pair Foods: Pair carbohydrates with protein and healthy fat to sluggish the absorption of glucose.

3. Regular Exercise

Stay Active:

- Routine: Aim for at least one hundred fifty minutes of slight cardio exercise in line with week, along with on foot, cycling, or swimming.

- Strength Training: Include resistance schooling sporting events at least two times a week to enhance insulin sensitivity and construct muscle.

Monitor During Exercise:

Check Levels: Monitor your blood sugar earlier than, for the duration of, and after workout to apprehend how bodily hobby impacts your levels.

Carry Snacks: Keep fast appearing carbohydrates, like glucose pills or juice, reachable in case of low blood sugar at some point of exercising.

4. Medication Management

Follow Prescriptions:

- Take as Directed: Take your diabetes medicinal drugs or insulin as prescribed by using your healthcare provider.

- Adjust as Needed: Work with your healthcare crew to adjust dosages based to your blood sugar readings and any adjustments in your ordinary or health popularity.

4. Exercise and Nutrition

How bodily pastime influences blood sugar.

Physical hobby has a enormous effect on blood sugar levels, and know how this relationship is critical for dealing with diabetes effectively.

Immediate Effects of Physical Activity

1. Lowering Blood Sugar:

● 	Increased Insulin Sensitivity: Exercise enhances your cells' sensitivity to insulin, permitting them to use to be had insulin greater efficaciously to take in glucose from the bloodstream.

● 	Glucose Utilization: During bodily activity, muscle tissue use glucose for power, which can decrease blood sugar stages.

2. Temporary Increases:

● 	High Intensity Exercise: Intense exercise, inclusive of sprinting or heavy lifting, can initially purpose a transient rise in blood sugar due to the release of pressure hormones like adrenaline. However, this impact is normally quick lived.

Long Term Benefits

1. Improved Insulin Sensitivity:

- Regular exercising facilitates improve insulin sensitivity over time, making it easier to maintain wholesome blood sugar levels and reduce insulin resistance.

2. Weight Management:

Physical activity enables with weight control, that's critical for controlling blood sugar degrees. Being obese can boom insulin resistance, making blood sugar management more difficult.

3. Reduced Risk of Complications:

Regular exercise allows decrease the danger of cardiovascular ailment, high blood pressure, and different complications associated with diabetes.

MEAL MAKING PLANS ROUND EXERCISE.

Meal making plans around exercise is vital for handling blood sugar tiers and maximizing the blessings of physical hobby for individuals with diabetes.

Pre Exercise Meal Planning

Timing:

1three Hours Before Exercise: Aim to eat a balanced meal 1three hours before exercise to offer sustained strength and stabilize blood sugar levels.

MEAL COMPOSITION:

Carbohydrates: Include complicated carbohydrates like whole grains, end result, or starchy veggies for regular power release.

Protein: Add lean protein resources such as bird, fish, tofu, or legumes to help muscle function and healing.

Fats: Include wholesome fat like avocado, nuts, or olive oil in mild amounts to provide lengthy lasting power.

Examples:

- Breakfast: Whole grain toast with avocado and scrambled eggs.

- Lunch/Dinner: Grilled chicken, quinoa, and roasted vegetables.

- Snack: Greek yogurt with berries and a sprinkle of nuts.

During Exercise

Duration and Intensity:

- Short Duration (<1 hour): Generally, no additional food is needed if the exercise is less than an hour and of moderate intensity.

- Long Duration (>1 hour) or High Intensity: Consider consuming a small amount of speedy performing carbohydrates to preserve electricity tiers and save you low blood sugar.